Recharge Your Immune System

8 Simple Steps to a Healthier and Longer Life

Table of Contents

Introduction

Everyone has a shot at living a healthy and long life. However, many people die prematurely because of certain factors in their life. These may include unexpected accidents or illnesses. Accidents are sometimes unavoidable, but illnesses can be avoided.

Our immune system keeps us healthy. If the immune system doesn't function well, you will have higher chances of getting sick. And we're not just talking about a common cold or a fever. The illnesses could be severe such as cancer.

That's why keeping the immune system healthy and in tip-top condition at all times is crucial to living a long and healthy life. Your immune system fights viruses and bacteria that can affect every part of your body.

In this book, you'll find out that it's easy to keep your immune system healthy. With these eight simple steps, you'll be living a life free from worry you could acquire a deadly disease.

You don't need any special skills. Each step includes a guide on how to do them successfully. All you need is have the will power and determination to change your life for the better since most of the things on the list involve lifestyle changes.

If you're ready to face a long and happy life and scrap the unhealthy lifestyle you're living, then be ready to do to the eight simple steps for a healthier immune system.

Chapter 1: The Importance of the Immune System

The immune system is your body's defense force. It protects your body from different bacteria and viruses. This is one reason the immune system must always be in tip-top shape.

Your body's immune system can recognize the difference between your cells and foreign cells. This lets the immune system destroy the cells that would be harmful to your health.

It comprises white blood cells (leukocytes), and there are different types. There are two main types of leukocytes – phagocytes and lymphocytes.

The phagocytes destroy harmful cells. The lymphocytes also help in destroying the cells, but they also "remember" the cells the immune system destroys.

The neutrophil, a phagocyte subtype, is often what doctors check in blood tests to see if the body can fight off diseases. Other phagocyte subtypes make sure the body can react and respond to foreign cells.

The two types of lymphocytes, the T and B lymphocytes, work hand in hand. The lymphocytes check the bone marrow and may turn into B lymphocytes. The cells could also go into the thymus gland and become T lymphocytes.

The B lymphocytes find the targets and lock the harmful cells. The T lymphocytes would then destroy harmful cells the B cells find.

Without the immune system, you'd probably be sick almost every time.

Once the body fights off a harmful cell, the immune system remembers it. So, the next time the same foreign cell would enter the body, the immune system would be ready with antibodies to prevent you getting the same illness.

The antibodies can also produce a different organism by neutralizing toxins. They can also activate immune system proteins that help kill viruses, bacteria, and even infected cells.

Chapter 2: The Consequences of a Weak Immune System

You already know what the immune system does for the body. It's also clear that having a weak immune system can be dangerous.

Some people may think that a weak immune system would result in regular cold and cough attacks. That may be a possibility, but there are far worse effects.

Effects of a Weak Immune System

A strong immune system will keep you healthy and away from harmful illnesses. If you don't take care of your immune system, you will catch more bacterial and viral infections easily than other people. This will affect your health and your entire life.

Imagine constantly battling colds, coughs, and fevers almost every time while you need to go to school or work regularly.

This is just the lighter case of a weak immune system. Sometimes, people get cancer and/or other severe health issues.

Primary and Secondary Immunodeficiencies

For unlucky people, they can inherit immunodeficiency from their parents' genes. This is called primary immunodeficiency.

This disorder impairs the immune system fully or partially. People with primary immunodeficiency are more susceptible to cancer and other severe illnesses at an early stage of their lives.

Treatments for primary immunodeficiency include stem cell and bone marrow transplantations, immunoglobin replacement, taking maintenance antibiotics, and some types of gene therapy.

Secondary immunodeficiency is acquired through various environmental factors. These may include severe burns, chemotherapy, HIV, and malnutrition.

Certain conditions may harm and attack the cells in your immune system, causing it to malfunction.

People of any age group are at risk of secondary immunodeficiency. The treatment may solely depend on the underlying cause of the immunodeficiency.

For example, HIV-caused immunodeficiency would need antiretroviral therapy, which stops the virus from multiplying. It would also help strengthen the immune system.

Cancer Treatments and the Immune System

While a completely shut off or weak immune system can cause cancer, the treatment for cancer can weaken the immune system more.

The most commonly used cancer treatment is chemotherapy. It involves strong medicine injected into your bloodstream to kill off cancer cells. However, the medicine is too strong that it harms the immune system as well.

The medicine would damage the bone marrow, making blood cell and platelet production weaker. It impacts the white blood cells or leukocytes more than the others. When there are insufficient leukocytes in your body, you'll be more prone to illnesses.

People undergoing chemotherapy also take other medications aside from chemotherapy medicine. This is also a factor that weakens the immune system.

Another factor would be the mental stress and depression that's common in cancer patients. It can lead to severe mental and emotional distress, which can harm the immune system more.

Sometimes, people choose other cancer treatments that don't include harmful medications. If the cancerous tumors aren't near the bones, radiation may be a better option. But radiation treatment directed to the bones can be more harmful to the immune system than chemotherapy.

Chapter 3: A Stronger Immune System for a Longer, Better Life

When you have a weak immune system, you risk not only your physical health. You also risk your mental state, your career, and your family among all others.

It keeps you from functioning as a productive human being. And the saddest part of having a weak immune system is your life span may shorten.

The Immune System of Elderly People

The immune system is your body's defense against all kinds of illnesses. Keeping it strong will help you maintain a longer and better life.

But as we age, our immune system slowly fades. That's why many elderly people develop different illnesses. Usually, the body's immune system would naturally fail at 65. Still, there are various ways to help keep it strong even at the later stage of your life.

In the entire world, Japanese people have the longest life span. Now, there are over 70,000 Japanese people aged 100 and above.

Their longevity and good health conditions may come from their strong immune systems. And it's not because they're lucky. Their lifestyle is one of the main reasons their immune systems are stronger than most people, which leads to a longer life.

Start Strengthening your Immune System Early

Most secondary immunodeficiencies begin with an unhealthy lifestyle that starts from an early age.

People in their younger years often take their health for granted; drinking, smoking, and using illegal substances – all of these could affect a person's immune system.

If a person continues to live an unhealthy lifestyle, the immune systems could weaken. This will lead to a shorter life span because you would pick up different illnesses. And as stated in the previous chapter, illnesses can lead to a weak immune system.

Parents should also take care of children's immune systems. Infants and toddlers are susceptible to diseases. Despite acquiring antibodies from their mothers during pregnancy and breastfeeding, their immune systems have no "memory" of many kinds of harmful cells.

During a person's early years as a baby, vaccines are often given to prevent fatal diseases. These vaccines help a baby's immune system to be ready if illnesses like polio or hepatitis strike.

Vaccines aren't used to completely block the diseases. Instead, it gives signals to the immune system about the disease and lets the cells remember them. Once the diseases hit a child, the immune system is ready to defend the body from the viruses.

Some people believe that vaccines can be harmful. However, there is no clear scientific evidence that can prove that vaccines can cause autism or other illnesses. Sadly, some parents don't give their children the vaccines they need. This leads to serious health issues later in the children's lives.

Vaccination is the first line of defense for any person's immune system. If your parents didn't give you the basic vaccines as a baby, consult a doctor and get yourself checked.

Chapter 4: Invest Time in Your Health Following 8 Simple Steps

If you've lived an unhealthy life of vices and junk food, it's not too late. You can still steer your ship towards a healthier lifestyle by following eight simple steps.

As you read through this book, you'll find out that strengthening your immune system only requires simple lifestyle changes.

It's not an easy task at first. You may find some changes time-consuming and difficult if your lifestyle is totally the opposite of a healthy one. But it'll all be worth the effort once you feel drastic improvement in your overall wellbeing.

Here are the eight steps for a stronger immune system.

Step 1 - Utilize the Benefits of CBD Oil

Step 2 - Be Wise and Use Bee Products

Step 3 - Drink Ginseng Tea

Step 4 - Hydrate, Hydrate, Hydrate

Step 5 - Pour Cold Water on Yourself -- Literally

Step 6 - Clear Your Mind through Meditation

Step 7 - Munch on a Lot of Fruits and Vegetables

Step 8 - Get Up and Move

Continue reading through the other chapters to know more about the steps. You'll also find tips on how to achieve with ease.

Chapter 5: Step 1 – Utilize the Benefits of CBD Oil

CBD oil – this has been creating noise in the medical field. Many people have tried using CBD to improve different health conditions.

Here's a simple understanding of how the CBD oil works in improving the immune system.

Your body contains the endocannabinoid system. This is a system that sends signals throughout the body to help it function properly.

The main benefit of CBD in helping the immune system is its anti-inflammatory properties. Inflammation causes a lot of autoimmune diseases. The CBD taps into the endocannabinoid system through special receptors. Through this, the body would respond by reducing inflammation.

CBD not only strengthens the immune system. It also calms down a hyperactive immune system. Hyperactive immune systems are as harmful as an immunodeficiency. It can damage your central nervous system – destroying scar tissues and fibers.

With an optimized immune system, you'd less likely acquire cancer. Cancer creates an inability for damaged cells to "remember" that they should self-regulate. This causes the damaged cells to multiply and spread in the body. CBD will help in inhibiting the spread of the damaged cells.

Choosing a CBD Oil Product

There are many types of CBD oil products you can take for your immune system. You may choose depending on your preference and lifestyle.

- CBD oil

- CBD tinctures

- CBD edibles (CBD-infused food products)

- CBD oil capsules

- CBD vape oil

Among the list, CBD oils and tinctures are the most popular and best to use. They have concentrated CBD.

If you're worried you'll get "high," get a CBD product without THC and hemp-based. THC is the cannabinoid that comes from the marijuana plant that gives people psychoactive effects.

CBD from hemp plants is often used for many CBD oil and tincture products. You'll find all the information from the seller's product description.

Note the CBD content of the product you're buying. The concentration may differ to give people choices.

For example, a 60ml bottle of CBD oil may contain 5,000 mg of CBD. This gives you 83.3 mg of CBD per ml of oil. Others may have a lower concentration like a 60ml bottle with 2,500 mg of CBD.

For beginners, CBD oil with low CBD content is best. This gives you room to adjust your dosage until you feel the effects.

CBD oil vs CBD tincture

CBD tinctures are more potent than CBD oils. Tinctures contain alcohol which acts as its solvent. Some people use tinctures because they want to infuse their drinks and foods with CBD.

If you prefer to take CBD directly into your mouth, take CBD oil. CBD tinctures may have a certain taste that not many people like when taken orally. CBD oil is tasteless, so it's much more tolerable.

CBD edibles

CBD edibles are basically food with CBD. Eating CBD edibles is an enjoyable way to take CBD, and you usually won't notice the

CBD in them. They are often sweet treats like candy bars and cookies.

The downside of this is that some edibles are high in sugar. There are sugar-free options, though.

More often, the packaging of the CBD edibles would include the CBD content per serving for easy dosing.

CBD oil capsules

You can also take CBD oil in capsule form. They're created by encapsulating CBD oil in soft-gel capsules, and they already have a specific dosage per capsule. You only need to take them like any other supplement.

CBD vape oil

If you're already vaping, you can use CBD vape oil as a replacement for your usual product. Using this product will let you inhale CBD into your system. You don't need to force yourself to vape if you're not into it. Just stick with the other CBD products listed above.

Taking CBD Oil for Immune System Maintenance

The CBD dosage would depend on your needs. If you have an existing condition, you may take an average or high dosage. Let's focus on CBD oil since it's the most common CBD product that will give you the best effects.

Before taking it, you have to compute how much CBD oil you should take. It would depend on your body weight and how potent you want the effects to be.

Now, you have to get CBD oil that will give you the right dose of CBD for every drop. Usually, one drop is equal to 1 ml, most CBD oil bottles already have a dropper included, so you won't have a difficult time.

Take a few drops every day distributed throughout your day. You could take your dosage 1-4 times daily, depending on your current condition. You can always ask a doctor for advice about taking CBD as a supplement.

How to Take CBD Oil

The best way to take CBD oil is by dropping it under your tongue. This is called sublingual administration.

Drop your dosage under the tongue and hold it there for about 60 seconds before swallowing. Do so every time you take CBD oil. This method can send the CBD into your system faster than digesting capsules or edibles.

If you're bothered by the taste or feel of the oil in your mouth, simply wash it down with a glass of water.

If you take CBD oil regularly, your body should function properly. It may also promote better sleep, which is another factor in keeping a healthy body. With enough sleep, your body can rest, relax, and repair itself properly.

Chapter 6: Step 2 – Bee Immune with Bee Products

While you're taking CBD, also take bee products as a daily supplement. Natural products such as honey, royal jelly and propolis have numerous benefits for your immune system.

Let's discuss what each type of bee product can do for you.

Honey

Honey has antibacterial properties and it's a natural antioxidant. It can help you improve your digestive and immune systems.

The antioxidant content of honey is high, which makes it very effective in removing free radicals and toxins from your body.

It also has great effects on common illnesses such as throat and respiratory problems, sleep disorders, and heart diseases. When other health issues are cured using this natural remedy, your risks of a weakening immune system will lessen.

You can take this in many ways since it is a versatile food ingredient. But you may try drinking a glass of this simple cleansing tonic.

1. *1 cup of warm water*

2. *1 tablespoon of honey*

3. *Juice from half a lemon*

Combine these three ingredients together and drink before eating breakfast every day. This will help cleanse the digestive system and absorb the benefits of honey for your immune system effectively

Some even try to just take a spoonful of honey daily, which is a straightforward way of taking it. You may also add a clove of garlic to relieve throat problems.

However, you need to be aware that many honey products are not pure. Some manufacturers cheat by mixing other liquids with pure honey to lower costs. Some even label syrup as honey to profit.

Only get "raw honey" made by a reputable company or buy directly from your local honey farm.

Royal Jelly

Royal jelly is another product made by bees. It's what the queen bee and her young feed upon. Many people, even in the past, have used royal jelly to cure different physical and chronic illnesses.

There aren't many studies on the effects of royal jelly on the immune system. Still, some researchers suggest that the fatty acids and the major royal jelly protein (MRJP) of royal jelly have their benefits. These are believed to strengthen the body's antibacterial activity that could result in lower infection incidences and a stronger immune system.

Because of this, taking royal jelly every day may help the immune system to function more successfully.

You can get royal jelly in many forms. The most popular ones are in powder or capsule form. However, these may include filler ingredients.

Luckily, you can buy fresh royal jelly in the market. They may come in gel form usually packaged in jars. There is also freeze-dried royal jelly.

Begin by taking ¼ teaspoon of fresh royal jelly every morning. From there, you can increase the amount to ½ teaspoon to 1 teaspoon after a few weeks or days.

Royal jelly has a naturally bitter taste with a hint of sourness. Some people may not like it at first but then develop an acquired taste for it.

If it's your first time taking royal jelly and you can't tolerate bitterness, mix it up with raw honey. An equal mixture of 1 part royal jelly and 1 part honey will help with the taste. Also, you would also get benefits from both products simultaneously.

Propolis

Another product from bees that can improve your immune system is the propolis. Propolis comprises sticky gums and resins that bees collect from trees. The bees add antibacterial components to the gums and resins, resulting in propolis.

Bees use propolis to block holes when the beehive is damaged. They also use it as an antiseptic, which prevents diseases from penetrating the hive.

Traditionally, propolis is used to ward off viruses and infections, which leads to a stronger immune system. It's a natural anti-inflammatory substance that promotes the activity of phagocytes.

Raw propolis come in chunks. You can chew on them, extract the liquid from the resin, then swallow the entire chunk. However, some people complained this method can stain teeth. If you still prefer this method, it's best to take 2 chunks every day.

For an easier way to take propolis, you can try using capsules, liquids, or powder. These have been processed and ready to consume. Capsules would have a controlled dosage and powders can be mixed with food or drinks.

The best dosage for starters could be 70 mg or propolis every day. Still, you may start at a lower dosage and work your way up.

Pollen

Bee pollen is another product that helps enhance immunity and relieve other health issues.

The pollen is gathered by honeybees while they move from one flower to another. The pollen flakes from the flowers are gathered into a "basket" on the back legs of the bee. Then, these flakes combine with nectar, which creates granule forms of bee pollen.

There have been studies that support the advantages of bee pollen to the immune system. It was found that bee pollen contains antifungal, antiviral, and antimicrobial properties. These may aid the immune system in killing viruses and bacteria.

Bee pollen is a versatile supplement you can add in various foods like oatmeal and yogurt. Some companies grind them into powder or make them into capsules.

The recommended daily dosage for bee pollen is around 20g-40g. You can also give children bee pollen with a 15g dosage every day.

These are the amazing bee products that will help you *bee* healthy. A great thing with this is that you can mix them all up to get their benefits simultaneously. You can choose what kind of bee product will work best for you.

But a word of advice – consult your doctor before taking any bee products. Being allergic or sensitive to some components in honey and other bee products. It's best to ask your doctor first to avoid any complications.

Chapter 7: Step 3 – Drink Ginseng Tea

If you're familiar with Chinese medicine, you probably know what ginseng is. It's believed that the discovery of ginseng was 5,000 years ago in the Northern China mountains.

Before it became an herbal medicine, people used it as a food ingredient. After many years, documentation dated around 200BC revealed the beginning of ginseng used as herbal medicine. Since then, the news about the wondrous plant reached other countries and more people continued to study it.

Because of its rich history, today's researchers continue to study ginseng. They found all the answers to their questions on the qualities of ginseng and its amazing benefits.

Ginseng Effects on the Immune System

Many researchers found evidence that ginseng can strengthen the immune system. According to the studies, ginseng is an effective anti-inflammatory and antioxidant remedy. Also, studies found that ginseng helps to increase the phagocytic activity of the immune system.

It helps prevent illnesses that can weaken the immune system. It could be taken for diabetes, mental health issues, cancer and high blood pressure.

This could be the reason Asians continue to take ginseng as a supplement through their golden years.

Types of Ginseng

You can choose from the two main types of ginseng: American ginseng or Korean (Asian) ginseng. Though both beneficial for health, they have different effects on the body.

Korean or Asian ginseng is more expensive than American ginseng, and there's a good reason for it. It's believed to be the most effective among other ginseng types. It's also the best for enhancing the immune system because it regulates metabolism making cells more active.

American ginseng is somehow opposite to Korean ginseng. While Korean ginseng gives off a warm energy, American ginseng may give off a cool one. It's also great for improving cellular health and prevents fatigue.

There are also other types of ginseng, which are the Siberian, Brazilian, and Indian ginsengs. However, they're not considered "true ginseng." You can still reap health benefits from these plants, but they're not as potent at the main ginseng types.

How to Take Ginseng

You can take ginseng in different ways. You can eat it raw if you can tolerate its taste. You can try steaming it first to make it easier to chew.

Ginseng could also be made into delicious tea. Slice ginseng and let it sit in hot water and let it steep for few minutes. You can drink ginseng tea every day in the morning or afternoon.

You may also add fresh ginseng to food items like stir-fried vegetables or soup. It's best cooked with chicken. There are many chicken soup recipes with ginseng available on the internet.

For raw ginseng, the recommended dosage is about 1 g-2 g every day.

If using fresh ginseng is too inconvenient for you, you may find different types of ginseng products in the market. Some products include capsules, tablets, powders, and oil.

Ginseng extract is concentrated ginseng. You can take it orally before meals. This will let your body absorb ginseng better so you can experience its full benefits.

The recommended dosage for ginseng extract is between 200 mg-400 mg daily.

You can try using ginseng powder and mix it with hot water to make instant ginseng tea. Create smoothies with fruits, vegetables, and some ginseng powder.

It's also possible to add ginseng powder to recipes, including baked items. Some people even like to add ginseng powder to steamed rice.

For people who may not like the taste of ginseng even when mixed with foods or drinks, tablets and capsules are available. These are made with ginseng extracts or ground up ginseng root. The ginseng content for each tablet or capsule is usually on the packaging of the supplement.

It's best to start with lower doses and increase your dosage over time. This will let your body adjust to the new nutrients introduced to your system. It will also prevent sudden side effects from occurring.

Also, don't take ginseng at night. Ginseng might keep you awake at night. This is why it's best to take ginseng first thing in the morning or during teatime in the afternoon.

Remember to discontinue use if you experience any allergic reaction after taking ginseng.

Chapter 8: Step 4 – Hydrate, Hydrate, Hydrate

Some people underestimate the power of drinking water. Others may also disregard water and would drink flavored beverages like juices, soda, and coffee. However, a diet that's composed of such beverages can harm your immune system.

Drinking soda and other sugar-rich drinks can weaken the ability leukocytes to destroy germs.

A regular soda contains around eight tablespoons of sugar. This amount of sugar together with the sugar content from other foods you eat, reduces your immune system's ability to function well.

This is why diabetics or people with high blood sugar lose the ability to heal wounds. Their weak immune systems make them susceptible to severe diseases.

If your diet consists of flavored drinks, limit it or stop and drink more water.

The Positive Effect of Drinking Water

Drinking water hydrates your body, which is an important aspect of keeping your immune system strong. It benefits all the systems in your body to function optimally.

Let's break down all the reasons drinking water helps your immune system.

Oxygenates the blood

Blood carries oxygen to different parts of the body. If you don't have enough oxygen in the blood, your organs may not function well. This will result in different illnesses.

Water comprises hydrogen and oxygen, which can help increase the supply of oxygen in your blood. It also aids the blood to carry more nutrients to all parts of the body.

And when your muscles, organs, and other body parts function properly, your immune system would too.

Detoxifies the body

Drinking water can help your kidneys flush out toxins more effectively. Without enough water, the kidney won't function well, which will also lead to serious conditions.

Toxins can prevent the responses of the immune system. When this happens, the toxin build-up would likely harm the body.

Promotes lymph production

Your body contains *lymph*, a special fluid that spread leukocytes and nutrients to all body tissues. It also carries other cells of the immune system and aids in detoxifying the blood.

Water plays a big role in lymph production. If lymph levels are too low or absent in the body, the immune system cells can't travel throughout your body.

Helps the digestive system

Drinking enough water is a crucial part in your digestion. You need enough water so your digestive system can break down food properly.

You need to eat a healthy diet to keep your immune system strong. When the food is digested well, all the nutrients from the food you eat will reach your immune system.

Also, water prevents digestive illnesses such as constipation. People who drink water every day in adequate volumes keep their digestive systems healthy.

Improves sleep quality

Sleep deprivation causes harm to the immune system. It results in a decrease in cells and bodies that help fight infection.

Through proper hydration, your brain would produce enough chemicals that will induce sleep. Because of this, your immune system would be able to stay strong and healthy.

Don't Drink Just Any Kind of Water

Not all kinds of water are equal. You must be aware of your drinking water source and how it has been processed. However, getting enough water in your body is more vital than your water type preference.

There are many types, including spring, purified, mineral, and tap. Whatever you choose, just remember that you need uncontaminated water.

Some people are lucky to have water sources that provide clean drinking water. However, some parts of the world have no access to that. They are often forced to drink harmful water, which usually leads to illnesses. As long as your drinking water is clean, you will have no problems.

How Much Water Is Enough?

There have been many opinions regarding the accurate amounts of water a person must drink. You may have heard that everyone should drink eight glasses of water every day.

This could be wrong since eight glasses of water may be a lot for a child but not enough for a 6-foot tall man. It's more reasonable to base it on your body, daily activities, and living conditions.

Your water intake would increase if you're an active person who exercises or play sports regularly. Living in areas with a hot climate would also increase the need of water since perspiring a lot can easily make you dehydrated.

Living in a cooler climate and living an inactive lifestyle may require you to drink less water.

Drink Water Daily

Don't go through a day without drinking any water. A single day without it may already spell bad news for your health.

As you wake up in the morning, drink water. You may also make tea by boiling water and adding ginger.

If you like creating your own infused water, drink more plain water than the volume of infused water you drink.

Eating or drinking anything that's flavored will take a toll on your kidneys. Drinking plain water will prevent many kidney-related illnesses.

Chapter 9: Step 5 – Pour Cold Water on Yourself – Literally

If you've seen the "ice bucket challenges" on the Internet before, you may think that it's silly. But many people have actually been doing this for their health even a long time ago.

This is called "cold therapy." It includes immersing, pouring, or showering yourself with cold water.

Cold Therapy Effects on the Immune System

The immune system has a vessel network called the lymphatic system. This runs throughout your body, which cleanses all bacteria and wastes from the cells.

When the lymphatic system slows down or the lymph fluid becomes insufficient, toxins will build up. This will result in pains, colds, injections, and other diseases.

Cold therapy contracts the lymph vessels to pump the fluids flushing out the wastes. Then, the leukocytes attach and kill the wastes in the lymph fluid.

Cold water triggers the lymphatic system to function properly, which lets the immune system do its work efficiently. This keeps your body healthy.

It also helps improve blood circulation and reduces inflammation which are two factors that also affect the immune system. When blood flow is stimulated, the immune system cells can travel effectively through all parts of your body.

Different Cold Therapy Methods

Here are the methods to cold therapy and how to do them effectively.

Immersion

This method is best for athletes and other experienced active people. For cold therapy immersion, you'll need a bathtub filled with ice cold water.

Some people have a high tolerance against the cold and would handle submerging in cold water even naked. If you need to use some clothing, it'll be fine as well. The toes usually get cold quickly compared to any other body part. You may need to invest in some shoes made from wetsuit material to keep your toes warm.

Remember not to submerge yourself too long in the ice bath. For first-timers, 2-3 minutes of immersion is enough. It's best not to go over 10 minutes unless you have a doctor's approval.

The downside of this is that it's not really water-efficient. You'd be using a lot of water for this every time you do it. Also, making your own ice bath can take much of your time, plus the cleaning process after that.

Cold Shower

Another method of cold therapy is taking cold showers. During this method, you won't need to shower continuously in cold water.

Start with a warm shower. Then, switch to a cold shower for a short time, roughly around 1-2 minutes. Dry off quickly and put on warm clothes.

If you could handle cold showers directly, about 5 minutes would be enough. Put on warm clothes or a bathrobe right afterward.

Cold Water Dousing

Dousing may be the best option among the three. It's water-efficient and easy to do.

To do this, take a large bucket and fill it with cold water. You can go as cold as you can tolerate.

Stand in the shower and pour the contents of the bucket from your head down. This should be done fast. This is best done in the morning.

In some parts of the world, dousing is done outside surrounded by nature while barefoot. This gives you a powerful connection to nature, which affects not only your physical health but your mental health.

Afterward, wrap yourself with a warm towel and clothes. Without the preparation time, dousing would only last for a few minutes, which may be ideal even for people with busy, on-the-go lifestyles.

Cold Water Therapy Risks

While cold water therapy has benefits, be aware of its risks. Before trying out cold water therapy, you must ask for your doctor's advice first.

People with preexisting heart conditions could put their lives at risk with cold water therapy. This is because the body has a reflex to a sudden temperature drop. The body's reflex may cause you to breathe in sharply and faster. Your heart rate may increase significantly as well.

Cold water therapy may also harm some people who already have a weak immune system. That's why starting with a higher temperature while gradually decreasing for every session of the therapy would be ideal.

There are also some people susceptible to chilblains or painful sores. The chilblains are responses of the body to wet and cold weather conditions. If you get chilblains during winter, you may need to avoid cold water therapy or get your body's reaction solved first.

Chapter 10: Step 6 – Clear Your Mind through Meditation

Meditation, when practiced right, can definitely improve your overall health. It's a practice where people use techniques to train awareness and attention to achieve a stable mental and emotional state.

It has been used in ancient times and often related to religious beliefs. Different religions have developed various techniques and strategies of meditation. Their disciplines and beliefs vary, yet their goals are somehow similar – to achieve peace and happiness.

Meditation has many mental health benefits. Reducing stress and anxiety levels may be one of the best effects of meditation for the health. This may affect the immune system as well.

Stress Harms the Immune System

"How can a mental health problem affect my immune system?" you may ask. Based on some studies, the immunity of people who experience a lot of stress decreases at significant rates.

It's because your brain and your immune system have constant communication between each other. Any disruption in the brain like stress, anxiety, and depression can have negative effects on the immune system.

When you are continuously stressed, your brain signals your endocrine system. Then, the endocrine system would release hormones that can put pressure on the immune system.

Stress triggers chemical reactions in the body, which can decrease inflammation. However, the reactions would also decrease the immune system cells, especially the ones responsible for killing cancer.

When this happens, the risks of tumor growth and development, tissue damage, and infection rate increase.

The effects of stress accumulate in the body, which leads to sudden and serious health problems. Even activities you do every day could increase your susceptibility to illnesses and diseases.

If you suddenly fall ill with no clear reason or source, it could have rooted from stress and your failing immune system.

Meditation for Stress

Meditation takes practice. You can't perfect it on your first try. But once you've mastered the technique, it will do so many wonders for your health.

There are many meditation methods you can try. The important thing is to practice it every day. A 10-minute meditation session can lengthen your lifespan and improve your overall wellness.

Read through the different meditation techniques and choose one that will work for you.

Using Your Senses

For this method, you can use as many of your senses as you with. This includes your smell, touch, sight, and hearing. Here are ways to get ready for a meditation session.

1. Stay in a room or even a place outdoors, which makes you feel comfortable and relaxed.

2. Set up a diffuser and use essential oils for relaxation like lavender or rose. If you're outdoors, smell the fragrance surrounding you by taking deep and slow breaths.

3. Play light, musical pieces that can induce relaxation. Try avoiding songs with lyrics that can distract you. If your outdoors, listen to the rustling sounds of leaves and chirping birds.

4. Sit in a comfortable position that you can hold for 10 minutes. Touch the ground, grass, couch, or chair you're sitting on and feel it gently.

5. When you're outdoors, look around you and take in the beauty of your surroundings. If you're indoors, focus on something that's simple and easy on the eyes, such as a piece of artwork or simply look outside your window.

6. You can also try closing your eyes and imagine a place or situation that relaxes you. Usually, background music can help you achieve this. If the view of the ocean relaxes you, try playing some background audio of the sea.

This is usually done with a teacher or guide. Still, it's possible to do this on your own with some practice.

Mantra Meditation

For this technique, you would need to repeat calming thoughts, phrases, or words silently. This can help you prevent negative and distracting thoughts.

Om is just one example of a mantra that's been used by many people all around the world. It's a sacred syllable in Hinduism believed to be the sound of creation. You can find many Hindu mantra words and phrases which you can use.

You may also create your own mantra. There have been people sharing their own mantras online. You can also hire some mantra experts that will guide you with mantras they've created.

To make a personal mantra, focus on what stresses you out or something that distracts you. From there, create a positive affirmation.

For example, you hear gossips about you spreading in your workplace. You can use the affirmation, *"I know myself better than anyone else."* This could be your personal mantra to help you get through the stressful issue.

Once you've decided on what mantra you'll use, follow these steps:

1. Find a quiet place with dim lighting to help you concentrate better.

2. Traditional mantra meditation would require you to sit in a cross-legged position. But if you find this difficult, you can sit straight and comfortably on a chair. You may also do it lying down on your bed or on any surface as long you're comfortable. Avoid doing it while you're tired to prevent sleeping during the session.

3. Focus on your breathing, but don't force or control it. Take slow, deep breaths.

4. Chant your mantra silently or audibly. This will depend on you. Saying it out loud in a modulated and calm voice is usually better.

5. After some audible chanting, switch to silent chanting. You may continue audible chanting if you wish.

6. If you're always on-the-go, 10 minutes of mantra chanting can already do a lot for your health. But you can still do it longer if needed.

The trick with mantra chanting is that you do it whatever makes you comfortable. You shouldn't force your mind and body to do it if you don't want to.

Sometimes, you can also practice mantra chanting to calm yourself down when you're feeling stressed in the moment. Create different personal mantras for each situation that stresses you out. Close your eyes and silently chant while taking deep breaths.

Mindfulness Meditation

Unlike the other methods which lets your mind wander off, mindfulness meditation requires you to increase your awareness of the present moment.

During this session, focus on what you're experiencing at the moment, like breathing. You'll be able to observe your emotions and thoughts and let them through without judgment.

Follow these simple steps to practice mindful meditation:

1. Take a seat in a stable, solid spot such as a chair or bench.

2. Sit in a comfortable position when seated on the floor. If you're using a chair, the soles of your feet should be flat on the ground.

3. Sit straight, but not stiff. Make sure you're comfortable and don't force it.

4. Place your hands on the top of your legs while your upper arms rest at your sides.

5. Look at what's in front of you and slowly drop your gaze downward. There's no need to close your eyes. You can let your eyes perch what's in front of them and not focus on it.

6. Next, bring your attention to your breathing. Relax and feel every sensation you're feeling.

7. Focus more on your breath. Focus on every inhale and exhale. Pay attention to the sensation of air passing through your mouth and nose. Mind the movement of your chest and belly when you're breathing.

8. Once your focus wanders off, don't panic. You can let it slide for a few minutes. Then slowly get back into your meditation and focus on your breathing.

9. When you're done, gently look up and take some time to take in the environment around you. Notice your physical sensations, emotions, and thoughts. Pause, take

one final deep breath and think about your day positively.

Find a schedule to do every day for a few minutes. This is a simple meditation method that anyone can do without a guide.

You can also do meditations which involved physical activities such as Qi gong, yoga, and Tai chi. These meditations usually are done in classes or groups. Some people may find group meditations more effective than doing it alone. You can try this out with a family or friend.

However, you may need to ask help from professionals or experts to guide you, which costs money. Still, you can always quit the classes after some time and do what you learned on your own.

Remember to choose a meditation method that will work for you. Choose your setting, which makes you feel relaxed to meditate successfully. You can join meditation classes with groups of people or hire someone for a private session.

Meditating every day will help you manage your stress, which can eventually strengthen your immune system for improved overall health.

Chapter 11: Step 7 – Munch on a Lot of Fruits and Vegetables

You are what you eat. Eating a lot of unhealthy food would mean *you* are unhealthy.

Your diet plays a big part in your immune system's condition. Studies show that eating a lot of sugar-rich foods affects the performance of your immune system cells to kill harmful cells.

If you have an unhealthy diet, start eating more nutritious foods that would benefit your body.

Nutrients Your Immune System Needs

Your body needs certain nutrients to function well. Since everything else is connected to your immune system, keeping all parts of the body healthy is essential.

Here are the main nutrients you should get from your diet every day.

Protein

Protein provides your body the building blocks it needs to develop. And contrary to the common belief that it's only for muscles, every cell in your body actually needs protein.

Antibodies, hormones, and other substances in your body include protein.

Your body needs amino acids. While your body can create amino acids naturally, there are amino acids you can only get from food. Protein can provide various amino acids that your body needs.

Fats

Many people avoid fat since they're known to have bad effects to the body. However, this is not entirely true. Healthy fats are beneficial to your immune system.

According to studies, fat helps the body absorb nutrients, clot blood, and build cells among all other benefits. With fats, your immune system can keep its cells healthy and ready to defend your body.

Fat can also help balance your blood sugar levels which can lower the risk of diabetes. It's also an important nutrient to keep your heart and brain healthy. It also helps in decreasing inflammation which is good for your immune system.

Carbohydrates

Another nutrient that your body needs are carbohydrates. Carbs provide fuel to the body to prevent diseases.

They give you the energy to do physical tasks like exercising. And with enough carbs during these activities, your immune system strengthens and recovers.

When you have enough energy because of carbs, you can exercise continuously which impacts your overall health. You'll reduce stress, improve your heart health, and strengthen your respiratory system.

If all other parts of your body are at their optimal condition, your immune system won't get too much pressure. You'll also lessen your chances of getting chronic illnesses, which may harm your immunity.

Vitamins

The body needs about 13 vitamins to function properly and you can only get this either from supplements or the foods you eat.

Each vitamin has an important task. If you won't get enough of each vitamin, you may suffer from health problems. While you need to get all the essential vitamins from your diet, your immune system would benefit most from vitamins C, B6, and E.

The most important immunity booster you should get is vitamin C. If you lack in vitamin C, you make yourself more prone to acquiring diseases. Vitamin B6 supports the chemical reactions in your immune system. Vitamin E helps to detoxify the body from infections and bacteria.

Minerals

Minerals, like vitamins, have different types and you need each of them for a healthy body. Minerals help your body to build strong bones and teeth, regulate metabolism and prevent dehydration.

For your immune system, you may need folic acid, iron, and zinc. These minerals perform specific tasks to help improve your immunity.

Folic acid and iron are responsible for cell production and maintenance. The cells that would benefit from folic acid and iron include the cells in your immune system. Zinc aids the immune system in fighting off harmful cells.

Water

Water is an essential nutrient. Find the benefits of water to your immune system in Chapter 8 of this book

A Vegetable and Fruit-Rich Diet

You may think that all these nutrients seem too much to think about. But all you need to do for you to get the nutrients you need is to follow a healthy and balanced diet.

A balanced diet would give your body everything it needs to function properly. To start, plan your meals. Your diet should consist of food from the five main food groups.

- Vegetables

- Fruits

- Protein

- Dairy

- Grains

A balanced diet would depend on your lifestyle, activities, and health condition. It could be overwhelming to plan your diet on your own that's why some people hire nutritionists to do it for them.

Nutritionists could cost a lot of money, so take time to research and you'll be fine on your own.

If you're an athlete, you may need to eat a bigger portion of protein and grains. For working employees, you can eat balanced portions from the five food groups. If you have any food allergies, it should be obvious that you need to avoid certain foods.

But no matter your lifestyle, it's best to eat a bigger portion of fruits and vegetables. Besides the fact that they're packed with vitamins and minerals, they're also low in calories. They also have fiber, which can support the digestive system allowing you to absorb more nutrients from the food you eat.

If you're an avid snacker, replace your candy bars or potato chips with some fresh fruits and veggies. They're healthier options to sugar and sodium-filled snacks.

You'd need to eat a variety of fruits and vegetables. Here are some fruits and vegetables that can help boost the immune system.

1. Citrus fruits like oranges, lemons, and grapefruits. They're rich in vitamin C.

2. Papaya is another fruit that's loaded with vitamin C. A single papaya can give you about 220% vitamin C daily recommendation.

3. Kiwi is rich is folic acid and vitamin C. It also has potassium, and vitamin K, which helps other body parts to function properly.

4. Bell peppers also contain vitamin C. It actually has twice the vitamin C compared to a citrus fruit. It's also packed with beta carotene which is good for the skin and eyes.

5. Broccoli has high amounts of vitamin E, C, and A. It's also packed with fiber and antioxidants. It may be the healthiest vegetable you can eat. Just try to limit the cooking time or try eating it raw. Cooking can strip off the nutrients and vitamins in broccoli.

6. Garlic is a staple in cuisines around the world. Unlike the other foods on this list, the immune-boosting effects of garlic may come from a compound called allicin.

7. Spinach is rich in antioxidants, beta carotene, and vitamin C. All of these may help in making the immune system function better. Like broccoli, try to limit the cooking time. If done properly, you can also enhance the vitamin A content of spinach.

8. Ginger can be used in many dishes. It's good for reducing inflammation and nausea.

There are still other wonderful fruits and vegetables you can add to your diet. The important thing is to eat various kinds of these produce for a balanced diet.

Chapter 12: Step 8 – Get Up and Move

The last step for a healthy immune system is to be active. There may not be much research about the relation of exercising to the immune system, but there may be clear reasons how it could help.

Exercise has many health benefits. This includes stress and weight control, blood sugar management, and improvement of mental and heart health.

After exercising, you would likely feel better. The chain of good effects on the body will eventually lead to a healthier immune system.

A Sedentary Lifestyle Puts You at Risk

If you live an inactive or sedentary lifestyle, you may be putting your life at risk. It increases your risk to acquire cancer and mental health illnesses like stress, depression, and anxiety.

You'll be more susceptible to heart-related diseases and your weight may increase at unhealthy rates. Your skeletal muscle mass could decrease because of sitting for long hours every day.

Basically, without movement, your body wouldn't function properly. And when other parts of your body are at risk from chronic illnesses, your immune system will be greatly affected.

Too Much Exercising Can Also Be Bad

There have been studies about the immune system and intense physical activities. According to the studies, intense physical workouts can temporarily weaken the immune system.

It's not actually that bad. When the immune cells drop, your immune system produces TNF, a kind of protein. TNF boosts immunity, kills cancer cells, and reduces inflammation.

More intense activities would mean a longer time for your immune system to recover. That's why some professional athletes would sometimes acquire some illnesses after long days or months of training.

For common people, long and light activities or short and moderate exercises may be the best way to keep a healthy immune system. In this way, your immune system will only take a short time to recover, limiting your risks after you exercise.

Simple Exercises and Activities You Can Do

It's best to exercise every day. There are many kinds of exercises you can do, and you can even create your own routine to fit your lifestyle. Here are some of the simple exercises and activities you can do without help from a trainer.

1. **Long walks.** Walking can have both mental and physical benefits. With just 30 minutes of walking every day, you can already improve your cardiovascular health and reduce weight. If you can, try to walk for more than 30 minutes but less than an hour. It's best done in an area surrounded by nature.

2. **Running**. If you're up for something more challenging, running for 20 minutes can also have the same effects as taking long walks. If you cannot handle running, you can start brisk walking first.

3. **Stretching.** Stretches may seem easy and some may think that it does nothing for the body. But when done right, stretching can relax muscles, relieve pains, and manage stress. You can also try yoga, which is a more serious practice of stretches and try to do it every day.

4. **Skipping rope.** The repeated jumping action uses the abdominal muscles, legs, arms, and shoulders. Do this for about 10-20 minutes every day to get an overall workout.

5. **Quick circuit training.** A circuit training involves exercises done in 30 seconds to a few minutes. It could be a moderate to intense workout depending on the

exercises in the circuit training. You can include crunches, push-ups, jumping jacks, squats, and lifting in your circuit training.

Sometimes, your daily activities could already serve as your exercise. For example, cleaning your home. Cleaning serves as a physical activity that involves all parts of your body.

If you live near your workplace, try biking or walking instead of using your car. Most exercises can also be done at home. If you're a busy person, find time in the morning or night to do the exercises for a few minutes every day.

You'll probably have a difficult time at first. Your muscles may become sore after exercising, but this is due to your body adjusting to a new activity that stressed the muscles.

To avoid this, start with very light activities and gradually increase the intensity. The important thing is to do it every day regardless of the climate. If you suddenly fall ill with a common cold or fever, you can still exercise. However, lessen the intensity to simple stretches or just walking for a short time.

Before starting any exercise routine, consult your doctor first. You may have an existing health problem which will worsen with physical activities. Ask for your doctor's approval you can exercise and ask what kind of exercises you can do.

Conclusion

A stronger immune system would equate to a healthier and longer life. It's like making sure your doors have secured locks so criminals can't get inside your home.

As you have finished the book, you learned the eight steps you should follow every day starting today for a healthier immune system.

You don't need to strictly follow everything in each step. Use them as guidelines on how you should live your daily life.

Doing the eight steps won't immediately cure all your illnesses. It will take time and continuous lifestyle changes for the steps to take effect.

Cut out all your vices that could harm your immune system – excessive drinking, smoking, and drug abuse. No matter how healthy your food is or even if you exercise every day, if you don't remove the harmful habits you have, it may not help at all.

Also, it's more fun to do this with a friend or a family member. Why not ask someone you know to do the steps with you? You'll also feel so much better knowing you have influenced someone close to you to live a healthier lifestyle.

Now that you have all the information to be healthy, it's up to you to act on it. I hope you learned the importance of your immune system and how it can affect your health.

Thank you for reading this book, and we wish you a long and happy life.